Kettlebell Long Cycle

A Twelve Week, Progressive, Long Cycle Competition Training Program for Beginners

Designed and written by Douglas Seamans Jr

Owner and Head Instructor – PRIDE Conditioning
Certified Personal Trainer
World Kettlebell Club Certified Combat Athlete Specialist
World Kettlebell Club Licensed Fitness Trainer
World Kettlebell Club Rank 2 Long Cycle - 90kg Lifter – 20kg Kettlebells
American Kettlebell Alliance Rank 1 Long Cycle – 85kg Lifter – 24kg Kettlebells
American Kettlebell Alliance Rank 1 Long Cycle – 90+kg Lifter – 24kg Kettlebells

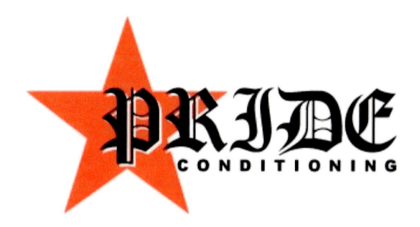

PRIDE Conditioning – 2139 McClintock Rd, Charlotte, NC 28205
704-334-3443

Please visit our website and blog for workouts, articles, training tips, motivation and recipes:
WWW.PRIDECONDITIONING.COM

Please visit our Youtube channel for videos on workouts and training tips:
http://www.youtube.com/user/PRIDECONDITIONING

Please train with a certified AKA or WKC Kettlebell trainer and become a part of the AKA or the WKC. You can find a trainer on both sites, you can also find competitions, training videos and kettlebells for purchase. Visit their sites here:
www.aka-sport.org
www.worldkettlebellclub.com

You can also find seminars and competition kettlebells for sale at Vulcan Strength
www.vulcanstrength.com

The information in this manual is copyrighted and is the sole legal property of PRIDE Conditioning and Douglas Seamans and is not to be shared or distributed without permission from the owner and publisher.

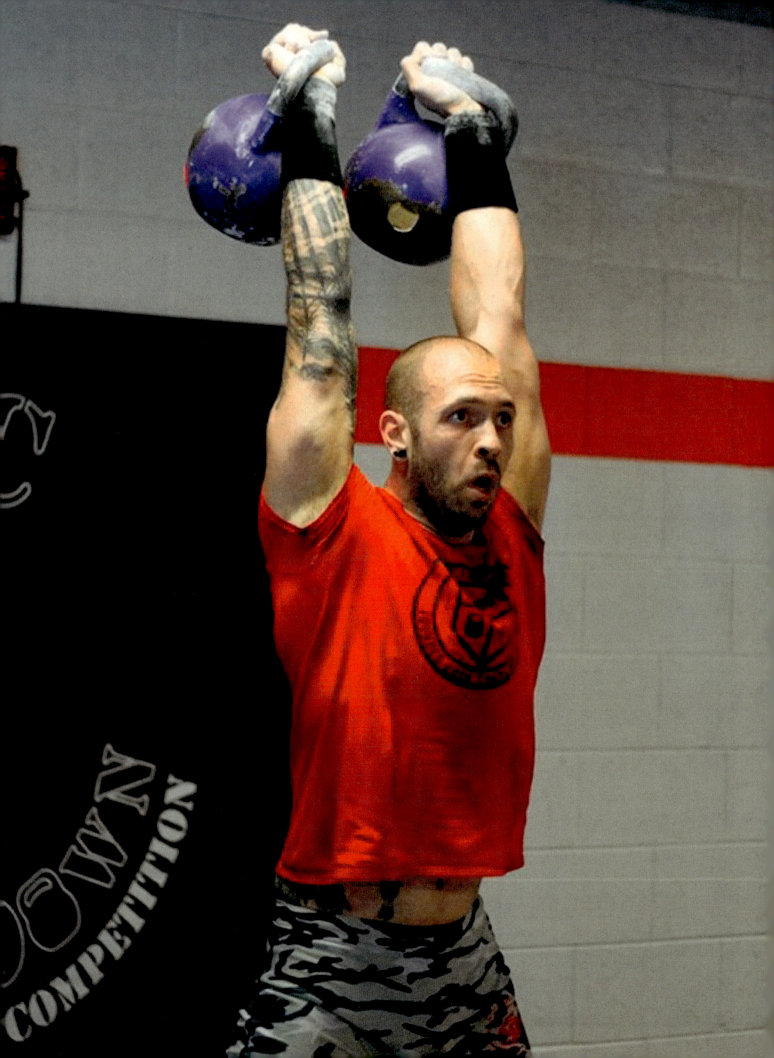

Disclaimer

Doug Seamans is not a doctor or a physician. Doug Seamans is not a Registered Dietician and is not a Nutritionist. Please consult with a physician and/or a dietician or nutritionist before proceeding with any diet and/or exercise program.

Assumption of Risk

Kettlebell training and competing in kettlebell lifting carries with it inherent risks, including but not limited to sever physical injury, permanent disability, paralysis and possibly death from cardiac arrest and/or dropping a kettlebell onto your body (including your neck and/or head). Doug Seamans and Pride Conditioning LLC, assume no responsibility for any and all injuries including death, inflicted on the user of this manual, onlookers, friends and family or any damage to property. (Note: There has never been a recorded death or paralysis in kettlebell sport competitions, statistically kettlebell sport lifting has the lowest rate of injury of all lifting sports. Kettlebell lifting is the safest lifting sport in the world, we just put this disclaimer in to cover our asses!)

Assumption of Knowledge

It is assumed that the user of this manual already has a basic knowledge of kettlebell lifting for sport and has proper lifting technique. It is also assumed that the user of this manual is an experienced kettlebell lifter and has been trained by a Certified Kettlebell Instructor on proper form, lifting technique, safety, breathing and how to do long cycle (clean & jerk) and any other kettlebell and non-kettlebell exercises in this manual. This is not a beginner's manual. This manual is not intended to train the user how to lift kettlebells or how to do long cycle. It assumed that the user already knows how to lift kettlebells. This manual is intended to instruct the user on a training schedule to prepare for a kettlebell long cycle competition.

Combat Sports

You will see "Combat Sport" listed in this program, combat sports such as Muay Thai, Jiu Jitsu, Wrestling, Boxing and MMA are an amazing way to get in a ton of cardio work, as well as endurance training of the shoulders, back, hips, legs and core. I personally train in Muay Thai and have been training in the TBA (Thai Boxing Association of the USA under Grandmaster "Chai" Sirisute) for over 6 years and it has been instrumental to my success in kettlebell training and competition. On top of the workout that you get from combat sport training, you will also gain greater flexibility and mobility and you will also improve your work ethic and mental strength.

Guarantee

I am so sure that this program will improve your lifting capacity that I am offering a 90-DAY MONEY BACK GUARANTEE! If after trying this program, you are unsatisfied with this product for any reason, simply send me a copy of your receipt and I will refund you your money. All you have to do is stick to this program and YOU WILL GET BETTER! Try it and if you have not improved or if you think this product is not worth what you paid for it, tell me why you want your money back and I will send you a refund.

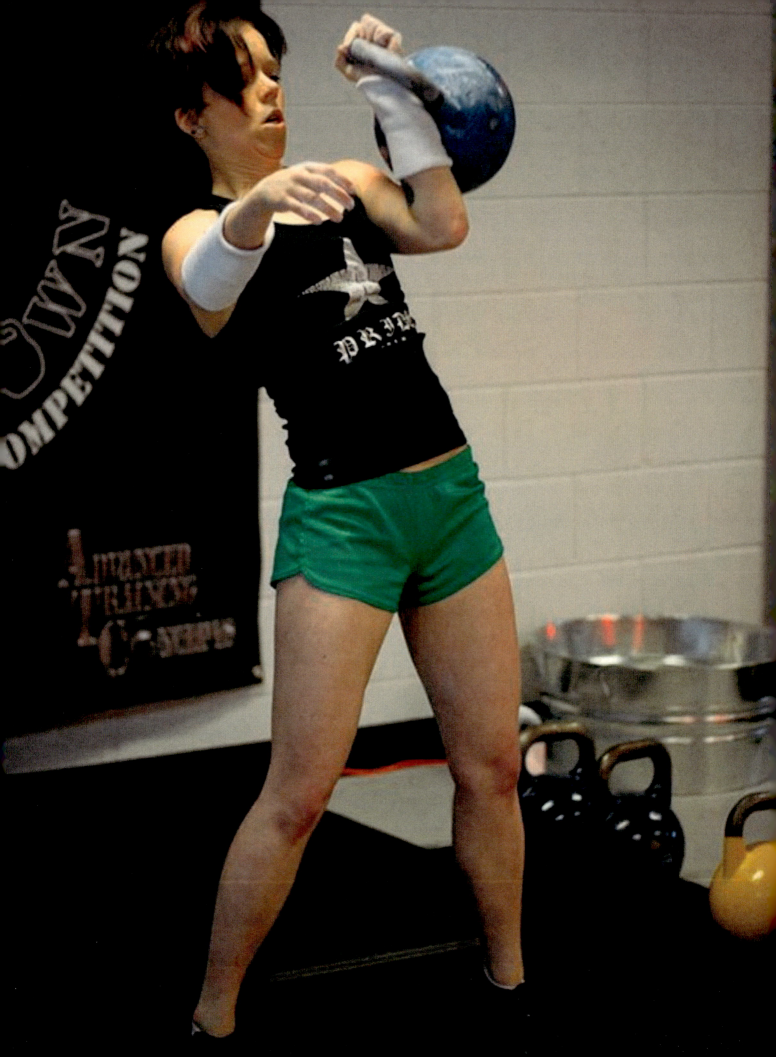

Dedication

This book is dedicated to the two most important people in my life: my wife and my mother. Without the love and support of these two people I would not be where I am today and I would not have become the person I am. Much love and many thanks to both of you for everything. Thank you to my momma, who, from an early age, told me I could do anything and truly made me believe that. Thank you to my wife, Lindsay, for sticking by me through all the rough times early in my fitness career and for believing that I could make this happen and thank you for all your design work and all your ideas, thank you for your love and for your support as we travel and lift heavy things.

I would also like to thank my coaches; Grandmaster Chai Sirisute, Ajarn Dick Harrell and Khun Kru Tim Sielaff (Muay Thai), Scott Shetler, Jay Trunzo, Chris Duffey and Cyrus Peterson (Kettlebell Instructors); thanks to all of you for all your time and energy and for keeping me focused and humble. Thanks to Cyrus for first introducing me to kettlebells and to kettlebell sport lifting, thanks to Scott for my second introduction to sport lifting, thanks to Jay for keeping me from losing my mind, and a huge thanks to Duffey for bringing me back from serious injury and taking my training to the next level. I would also like to thank one of my trainers from my childhood, Shihan Johnny Owens; thank you for starting my journey in the world of fitness and Martial Arts at such a young age and for instilling in me the respect, discipline and dedication that have helped me become the man I am today. I cannot write a book about kettlebell training and lifting and competing without thanking Valery Federenko for bringing kettlebells to the united States and showing us how to lift properly and safely; you have shown many of us a completely different way to workout, to improve our mental and physical strength and you have given many of us a profession and a way of life. Thank you.

Lastly, thank you to all of my clients, I do this for you, day after day, writing workouts, teaching proper form and technique, and motivating you to become better, stronger and faster. The success stories I receive from you, my clients and friends, are a huge motivation, so thank you for all your hard work.

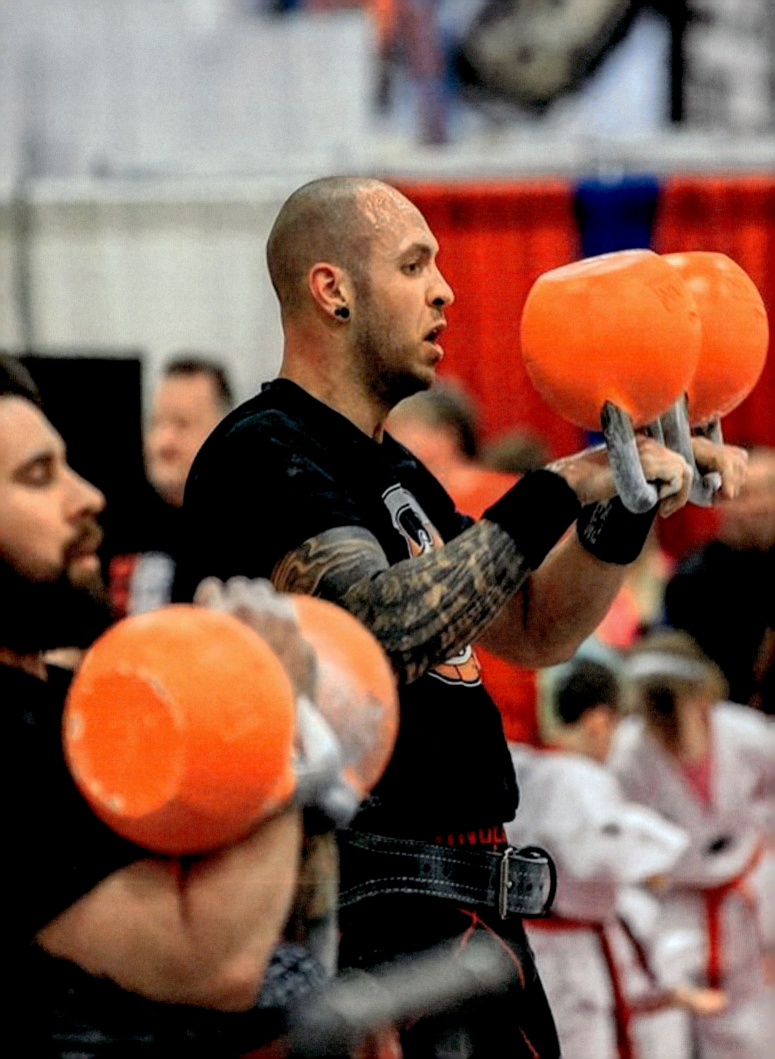

Introduction

So, you want to compete in a kettlebell competition? You want to do Long Cycle for 10 minutes? Want all your reps to count? Want to get cleaner, smoother, faster reps? Then this book is for you! In this manual, I have laid out a progressive 12 week training program for competing in a Long Cycle (LC) event. If you look closely and flip to the end of this program you will see that the program is actually 13 weeks; it is 12 weeks of progressive training and then one week of tapering and rest. This program will benefit everyone from newbies to the highly experienced, but it is truly designed for the beginner lifter going into their first competition. I will be releasing a more advanced program for stepping up to a new weight or for more advanced lifters.

While I am not the most experienced kettlebell lifter on the planet, nor am I the strongest or the fastest, the information I am going to share with you can be put to use and I guarantee it will help make you a better lifter. I have been lifting kettlebells for over 6 years and I have been dedicated to kettlebell sport, training and coaching for more than half that time. If you are training by yourself, this program will help guide you, but I highly recommend you seek a qualified, experienced and licensed kettlebell trainer to coach you, watch you, direct you, correct your mistakes and to motivate you. I also recommend you record all of your kettlebell training sessions on video and review them to look for areas where you can improve, from your breathing to your clean technique to your rack position to explosiveness to lockout. Even if you cannot find a coach within your city or within driving distance you can find a coach that will train you remotely by watching your videos and giving you critiques on your form and helping you with your programming.

I have attached a training schedule that you can print out and mark down your progress. This program is formatted for male lifters on double kettlebells, if you are a female, simply cut the times in half and put in a hand switch at the halfway mark. This program is 6 days a week; 3 days on the kettlebells and 3 days on GPP (General Physical Preparation) and SSP (Sport Specific Preparation) and some LS (Long Slow) cardio.

An important point in this program is the end of the first 4 weeks. At this time you should be able to make a 5:00 set at your competition weight. If by the end of the first 4 weeks you are not able to complete five minutes at your competition weight then you are probably not ready to compete on that heavy of a kettlebell. If you are not ready for that weight you have two choices; you can either drop down to the next weight or continue just doing the best you can and go to the competition to try and hit a time PR. If by the end of this program you cannot make the full ten minutes, it is ok, go to the comp and do your best. If your best in practice was six minutes and you make eight minutes at the comp then it is a win for you and a PR, congrats! Do not expect to win any records at your first comp, it really is you versus you, just go lift, do your best and have fun!

With that said, by the end of this program you should be able to make 10:00 on your competition weight, if it is your first competition. If you have already competed and you are stepping up to a new weight then you may need a longer program, but the information and program here can most certainly help you. Making the full 10:00 is goal number one, after you have reached that goal, then you can worry about how many reps you get in 10:00. A great lifter, coach and judge by the name of Mike Sherman once told Lindsay and me, "I cannot tell you how many times I won 1st place because the guy next to me put the bells down at 9:30

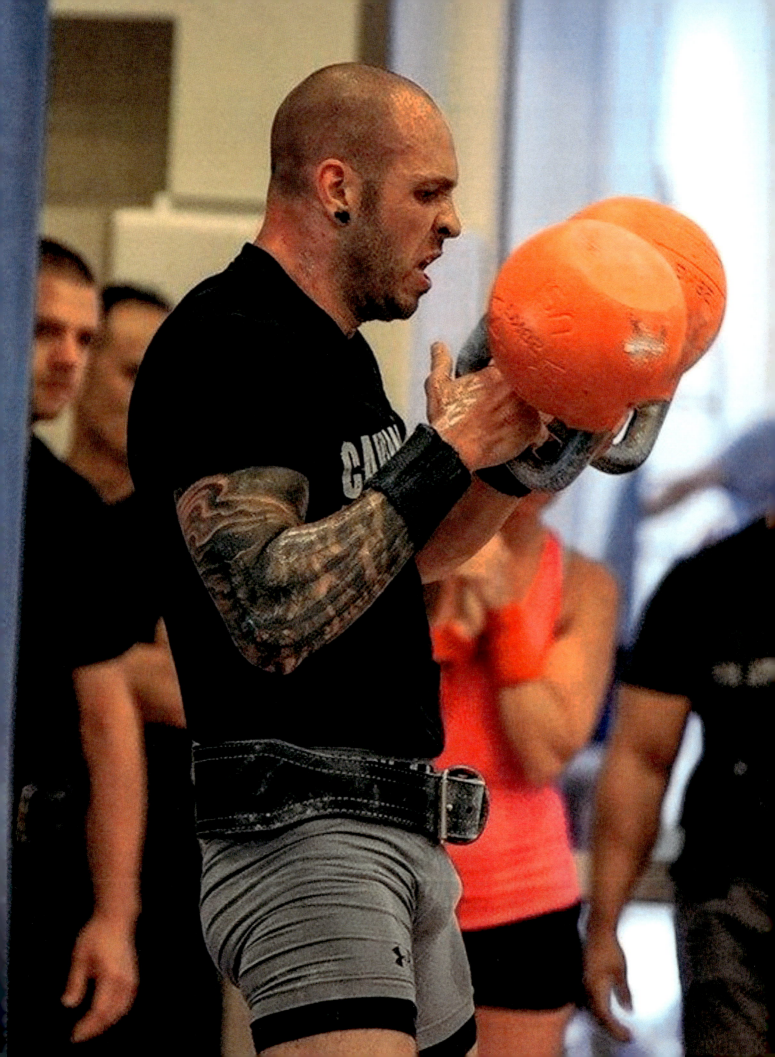

and I finished the last 30 seconds." Toughing out that last minute, that last 30 seconds, making one more rep than the lifter next to you is one of the keys to being successful in this sport. I recently tied for 2nd place at a competition because I toughed out the last ten seconds, made one more rep and the lifter next to me put the bells down with 20 seconds left, if he would had made one more rep I would have bumped to 3rd place. I won the AKA Nationals on 28kg Long Cycle because my competition put the bells down a little after the 7:00 mark. Try to make that 10:00 people, and have fun!

The key to your success is also the only thing holding you back from success, and that is you! You are the key, but you are also your own worst enemy. You have to believe in yourself, you have to believe that you can train hard, compete and succeed! Without believing in yourself and dedicating yourself to your training, you will not succeed. This program is a guide, it will show you what to do, when to do it and how to train properly, but without dedication this program is just a bunch of words. This program only works if you work and you work hard!

Now if you're ready to start training, let's get to work!

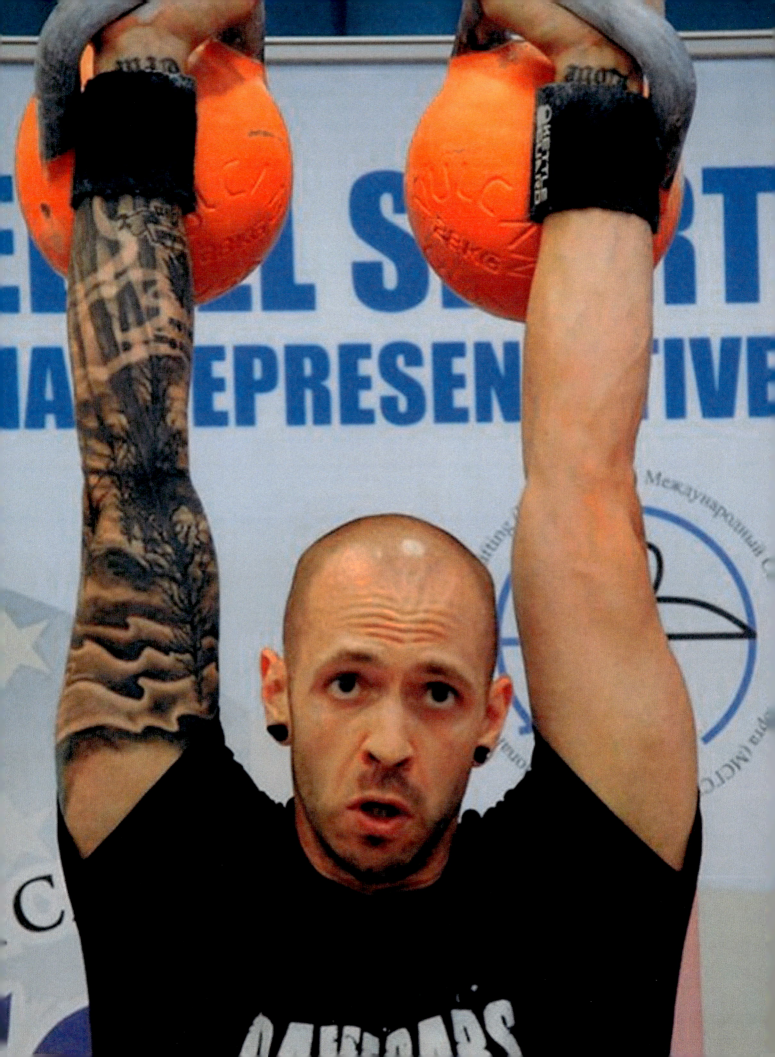

Fixation

Again, I am assuming you know how to do a clean and jerk, you know how to perform Long Cycle, so you must know about fixation. But do you really know? If you have competed in the WKC or you have sent in a ranking submission video or you have a certified WKC Trainer or Coach, then you should know all about fixation. As one of my trainers told me "the WKC is fixated on fixation". This is neither a good nor a bad thing. Fixation shows that you have control of the kettlebells, it shows that you are strong enough to lock them out and hold them and keep them from moving and you are not dropping them too fast from lockout. Fixation can destroy you, both mentally and physically. When you are first getting used to exactly how the WKC wants you to fixate and how long they want you to fixate overhead in lockout, it can drain you physically and it can frustrate you to no end. Trying to figure out why you are not fixating properly while competing can break your concentration and it can also cause you to lose reps and time, time you must make up by going through the bottom portion of your reps much faster than you want to, leaving little to no rest in the rack position. If you are competing in any other lifting organization they may not be as strict as the WKC on fixation, but you will still need good lockouts no matter which organization you are competing under, but beware the WKC is very strict on fixation. Also, if you are competing outside the United States, especially in Europe, Eastern Europe and Russia, no matter what governing body you are going to compete under, they will be very strict on fixation, and while it may look like other lifters are only locking out for one thousandth of a second, they are still locking out and fixating, their form and technique is that good.

If you are new to competing then you may be asking "what the hell is fixation?" Fixation is when you lock out the kettlebells overhead and they stop moving. The bells must pause, no movement, side to side, front to back, up and down - zero movement. The following terms are issues in lockout that will give a judge cause to no-count your reps:

- Bounce: when you put so much force into pushing the kettlebells up with your hips that they bounce at the top of your lockout. If this happens, you must take the time after they bounce to set your lockout and stop them from moving. To fix this you just need to tone it down a bit, only use as much energy as you need to, no more.
- Wobble: when your arm shakes in lockout. This usually happens when you are tired or if you cannot lockout your elbows straight due to poor flexibility or tight biceps. To fix this you need to improve your flexibility and your strength.
- Drift: when you lock the kettlebells out straight up overhead but they start to drift to the outside of your stance away from the centerline and you drop them from lockout before stopping them from moving. You need to work on keeping your arms straight and in the same position, staying close to the center line. Try keeping your biceps close to your head.
- Fast Drops: when you do not fixate long enough, you are putting the kettlebells overhead and straightening your arms but you are not leaving the bells up in lockout position long enough. The kettlebells do not need to stay up there forever, watch the masters, their lockout is fast, only a split second, but the bells make a notable pause, they stop moving and are then dropped. The simplest way to fix fast drops is to breathe, taking a breath overhead will help you relax and set your lockout.

- Alignment: when your arms are overhead, but they are forward of your head, not in line with your hips and the rest of your body. Improper alignment is usually easy to fix, simply stick your chest out and your butt out and think about bringing your elbows next to your ears.

I wish I could say that fixation is easy to learn but it is not. My advice to see what proper fixation looks like, is to watch videos of all the masters, Federenko, Denisov, Igor Morozov, Anton Anasenko, Denis Vasiliev, Sergey Rachinsky, Sergey Merkulin, American lifters like John Lesko and the infamous New Zealander Paul White and the ladies such as Surya, Ksenia, Melissa Swanson, Svitlana Krechyk, Jessica DiBiase, Lorna Kleidman and others, and to then video yourself and compare your form, technique and fixation to theirs. My next piece of advice, to fixate properly, is to relax and breathe. Relaxing overhead in lockout and going through a full breath cycle will help set your arms and shoulders in place and help stop the kettlebells from moving.

Alignment

Alignment is the relationship and position of your body with the kettlebell locked out overhead. In competition the judges not only look at your fixation, but they also check your alignment; if you are not aligned correctly, if you are leaning forward or back too far or your arms are not aligned with your hips and feet properly your reps will not count. In old school rules, proper alignment meant you generally had to have your biceps just behind your ears. Now, not everyone has this degree of mobility, most people cannot bring their arms into a perfectly straight position overhead, and if they can make them straight most cannot bring them close to their head or behind their ear. But this is how you need to look, even if you cannot get your form perfect now you still need to work on it over time, every set you need to work on that perfect alignment until it is...perfect.

Now, some judges and some lifting organizations are far more or less strict than others when it comes to alignment. At my first competition they were fairly strict when it came to alignment and the very next competition I went to they were not strict at all. Just get those arms straight, take a breath, and you'll be fine! Be sure to talk to your judge before you start your set if you have any major mobility issues that result in your lockout not being perfectly straight at the elbow or if your alignment at your ears and in line with your hips. As long as you perform your lockout and the bells pause overhead for a split second and do not move then you should have your reps counted. Even if your lockout is not perfectly straight, but you make your judge aware of your mobility issues, as long as you fixate they should count your reps. It is when you start doing fast drops or have major wobble or drift or shake that you will get no-counts.

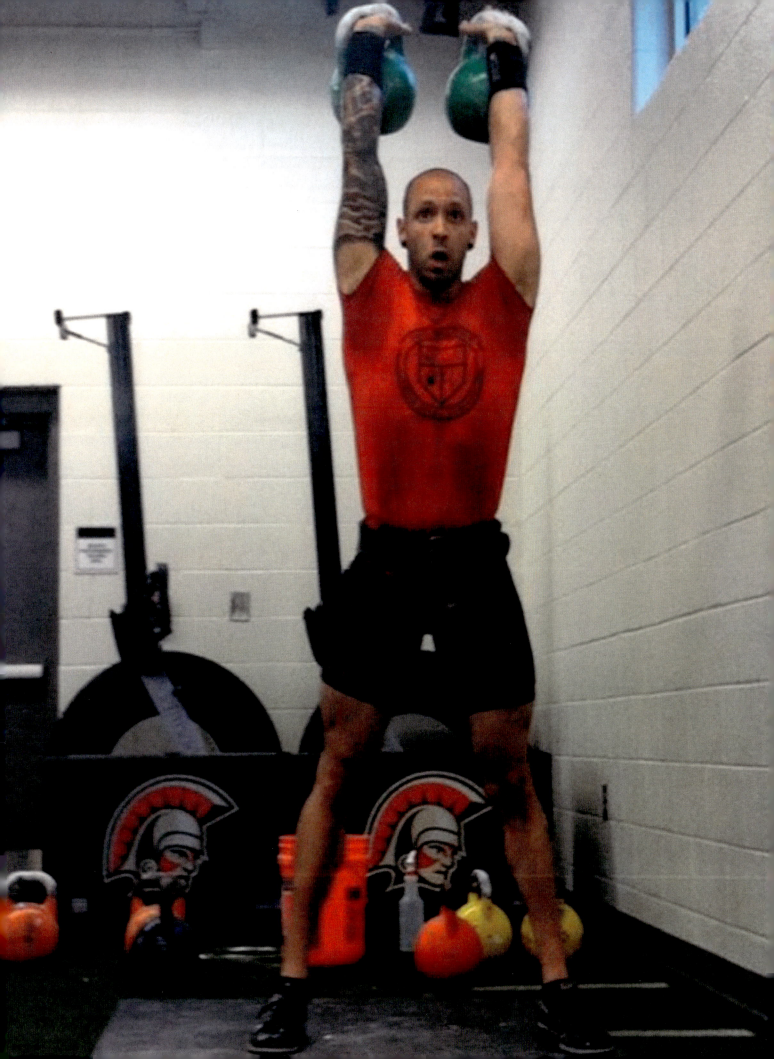

Blatant product endorsement here...

You will notice in many pictures I am wearing a set of wristguards. The only wristguards I will wear are also the only wristguards legally allowed in AKA or internationally in IUKL competitions are "Kettleguards". According to national and international rules your wrist guard must be no more than 10cm wide and no more than 25cm long and must be flexible in both directions. The "flexible in both directions" part is important as some other wristguards will only bend in one direction and they are therefore against the rules. The wristguards must be able to bend left to right and front to back and diagonally. Kettleguards are the only wrist guard on the market that meets all of these requirements. Not only do they meet the requirements, but you can choose different levels of protection by inserting 1 or 2 or up to 3 plastic pieces into each slot on the guard. You can purchase online through Amazon or straight from Kettleguards at their website www.kettleguard.com.

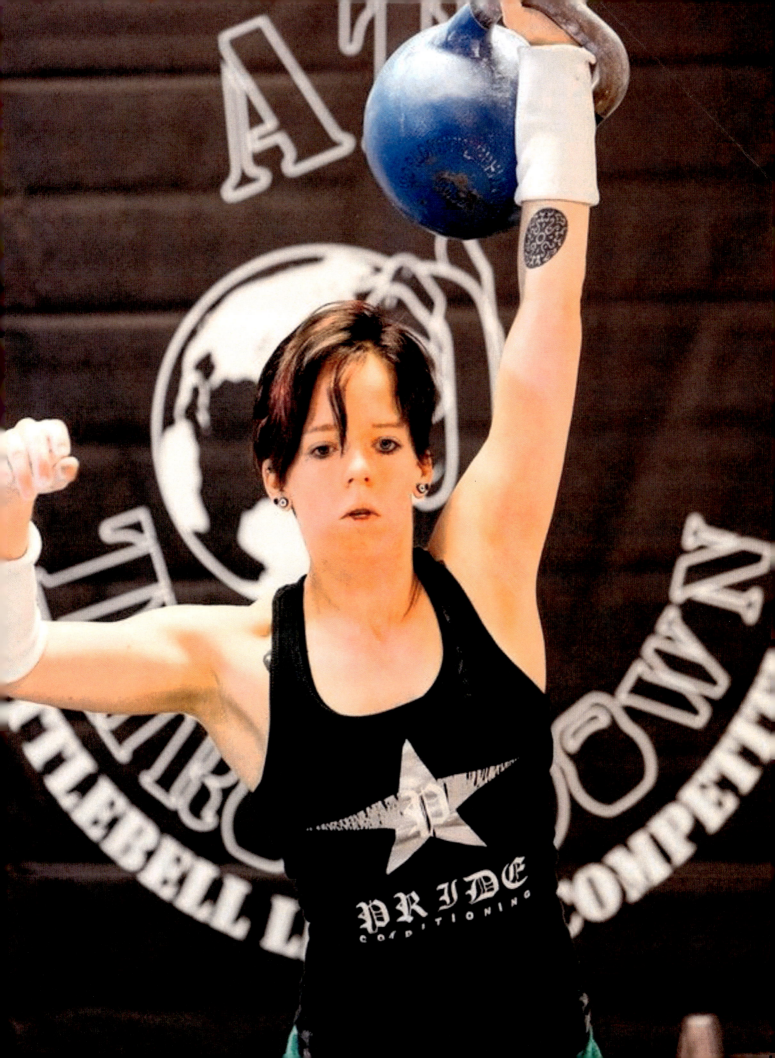

Warm Up

My warm up for long cycle training is almost always the same; 5:00 of either rowing, jumping rope or Airdyne, and I usually finish with 10-20 medium height box jumps to wake the legs up, but if my calves or something else is hurting I will switch it up. Also, I always go through a lot of dynamic movement work; high knee steps, goose steps, butt kicks, squats, squat thrusts, lots of arm circles and neck circles as well as shoulder opening drills with a piece of PVC pipe and then go for a quick 400 meter jog. I then stretch my hips, shoulders, legs, back and loosen up all my joints with simple rotation exercises. Then I warm up on the kettlebells, going down two to three weights from my competition weight and performing:

- 20 swings on each hand,
- 10 cleans on each hand,
- 10 snatches on each hand,
- 10 jerks on each hand, two weights down and then one weight down.

Warm up is finished up with 1:00 (usually 8 reps) of LC on doubles on lower weight, then another 1:00 LC doubles on the next weight up, focusing on explosion through the legs and hips and focusing on breathing. Before you start your set on your comp weight, push 5 reps on that weight so that when the bell rings and you pick that comp weight up you are not shocked by how heavy it is. When doing your warm up set of long cycle reps, truly focus on the movement and your breathing, and relax. After I have gone through my warm up work, I take a break for five minutes to mentally prepare for the workout, then I go through a set of 20 jerks without any weight, I focus on getting my butt down in order to lockout my arms and I focus on speed. All that for a 10-30 minute workout!

Foam Rolling and Static Stretching

I do not recommend any static stretching before the workout, I recommend static stretching and rolling after workout, pre-workout should be dynamic stretching. I (and many other trainers) believe that static stretching before a workout hinders performance by making your muscles and joints too lose and too relaxed. Some lifters, like my assistant trainer Matt Hooker, are extremely tight, they are in yoga everyday and if they do not stretch and roll before a workout they will fail miserably on that workout. if you are one of these people you need to find that knife's edge between stretching and rolling before to warm up to loosen up the muscles...and doing too much stretching and rolling which may be releasing lactic acid and wasting too much energy before your workout. You always want to stretch and roll after your workout is finished. Also, water and fluid consumption as well as your diet play a huge role in your muscle soreness and cramping. People who are in a constant state of dehydration because they do not intake enough fluids as well as people who eat a lot of food products containing dairy and gluten will experience more muscle fatigue, cramping, stomach issues, mucus in the throat and lungs as well as stiff joints. Please drink a lot of water before your workouts and throughout the day, eat a clean diet and get off foods filled with processed garbage, sugar, HFCS (high fructose corn syrup), wheat gluten and dairy products. Lastly, people who consume lots of processed white sugar will often experience muscle cramps in their legs, so if you don't want cramps, lay off the sugar and the white bread.

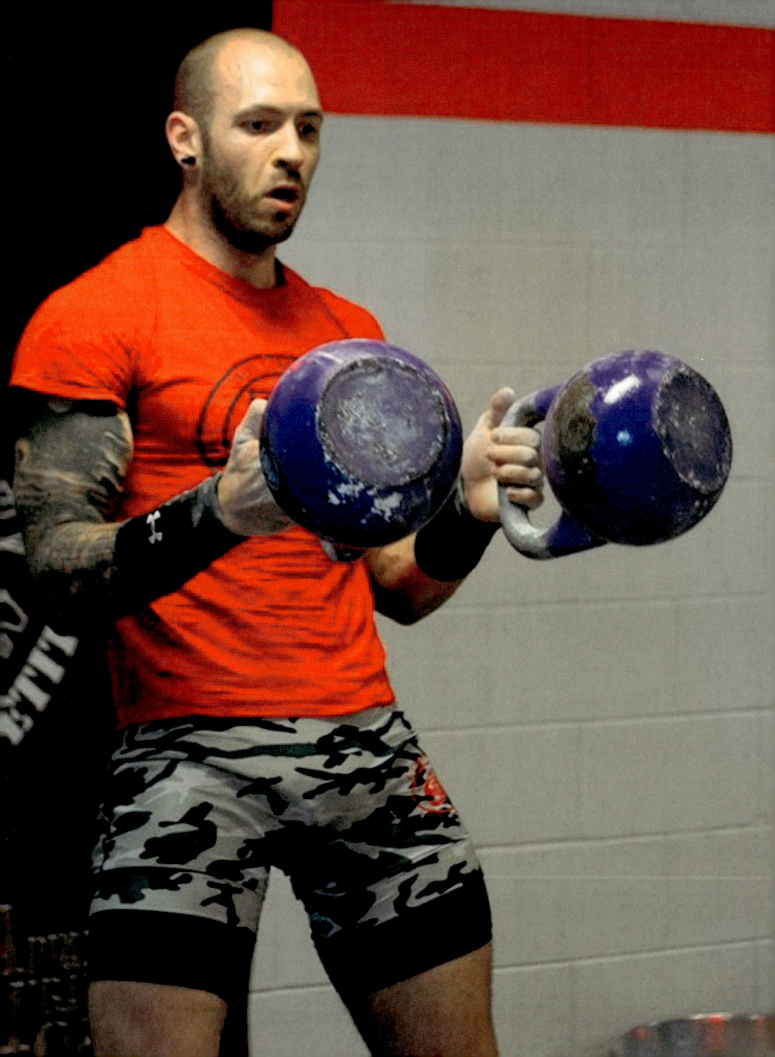

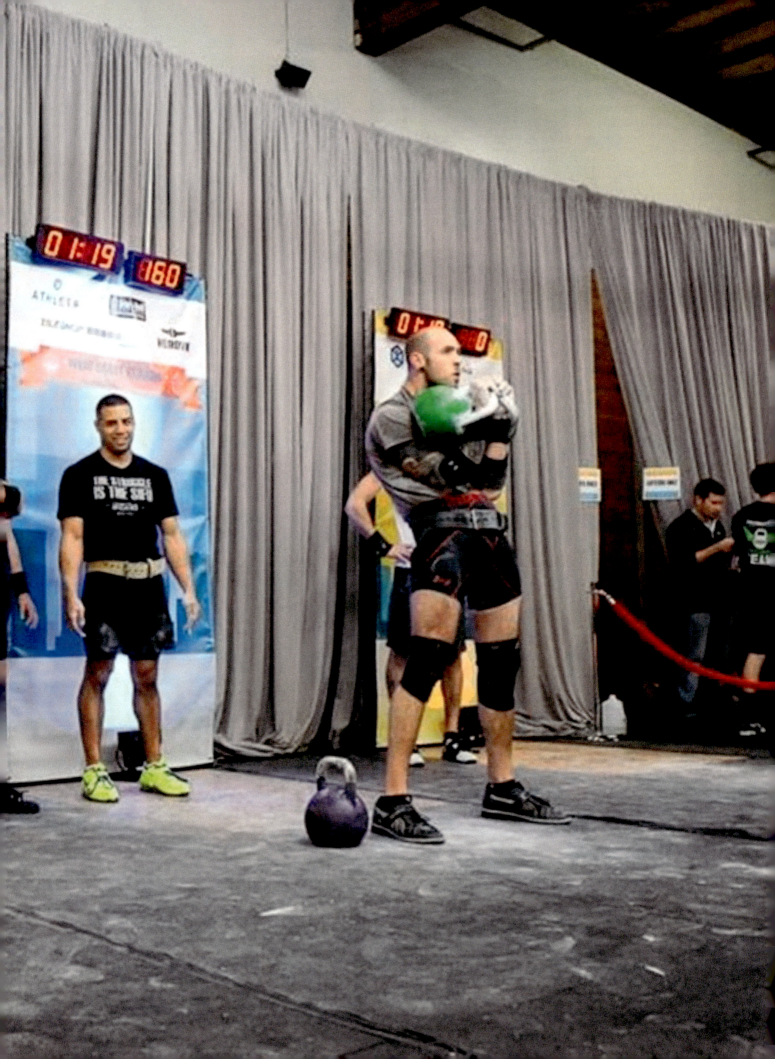

TWELVE WEEK LONG CYCLE TRAINING PROGRAM

Weeks 1-4

Monday
1 x 5:00 Long Cycle

(With competition weight. If this is your first competition you may need to work up to this. In this first three weeks just try your best to make 5:00. If this is your second comp you can go for 6:00. If you are stepping up to a heavier weight then do 4:00 your first 2 weeks and then 5:00 the 3rd and 4th week. Try to maintain 5rpm.)

5 Rounds:

10-15 Decline Push Ups
5-10 Pull Ups or Reverse (Suspension/TRX) Rows

Finish:

10:00 Row or Run
-OR-
Combat Sport: 5 x 3:00/1:00 rounds of Bag and/or pad or mitt work

Tuesday
5 Rounds Lifting:

5 Squats (Front or Back Squats, your preference)
10 Chin Ups
5 BB Deadlift
10 Skull Crushers or Band Pull Downs or Tricep Extensions or Skull Crushers

Finish: 20:00-30:00 bike ride or 10 x 1:00/0:20 intervals on Airdyne and Box Steps (20:00)

Wednesday
5 x 2:00/1:00 Rounds Long Cycle at 6-8rpm
(First two rounds with comp weight, next two rounds one step down, last round with two steps below competition weight. The goal here is decent speed, not quite a sprint but close. You still need to perform good lockouts and fixate properly, but you need to spend as little time in rack as possible.)

1 x 2:00 Jerks (One step below comp weight at 6rpm.)

5 Sets of:
5 BB Shoulder presses (take at least 60 second between sets)
0:30 Seated Grip Drill (on a bench, legs wide, back straight, two kettlebells, swing just a couple inches back and forth, between the legs, use a weight one step up from comp weight.)

10 x 1:00/0:15 Rounds of cardio interval work (running, jumping rope, bike, boxing, etc)

Thursday
Cardiac Development

3 x 3:00 x 3 sets (total work time is 27:00)
-Row
-Run
-AMRAP: 3 Burpees, 3 Jump Squats, 30 Mountain Climbers
There is no rest in this workout, your pace will be and should be slower!

Friday
6 x 1:00/0:30 Long Cycle Sprints (First 3 @ comp weight and 3 @ one step down. Try to maintain 6rpm.)

Lifting:
5 Sets
-5 BB Back Squats
-10 DB Curls
-10 Band Pull Downs or Rope Tricep Extensions

Finish:
3 Sets of 10 BB Quarter Squat Jumpers (with 2:00 rest between sets)
*It is important that you land soft! If you do not land soft the bar will hurt you!
*Do not string together your jumps, make each jump as high as possible, land soft, rest by standing up straight, make your dip just like your first dip on Long Cycle and explode!
*Use a weight 20%-25% heavier than what you will push in competition

Sprints:
10 x 20 Meter sprints with 0:30 rest between each sprint

Saturday
Lifting:

5 Sets
-5 Deadlifts
-10 DB Curls
-10 Skull Crushers
-5 BB Shoulder Press

2 x 5:00 Jump Rope or Boxing/Kickboxing or 10:00 Run or Row

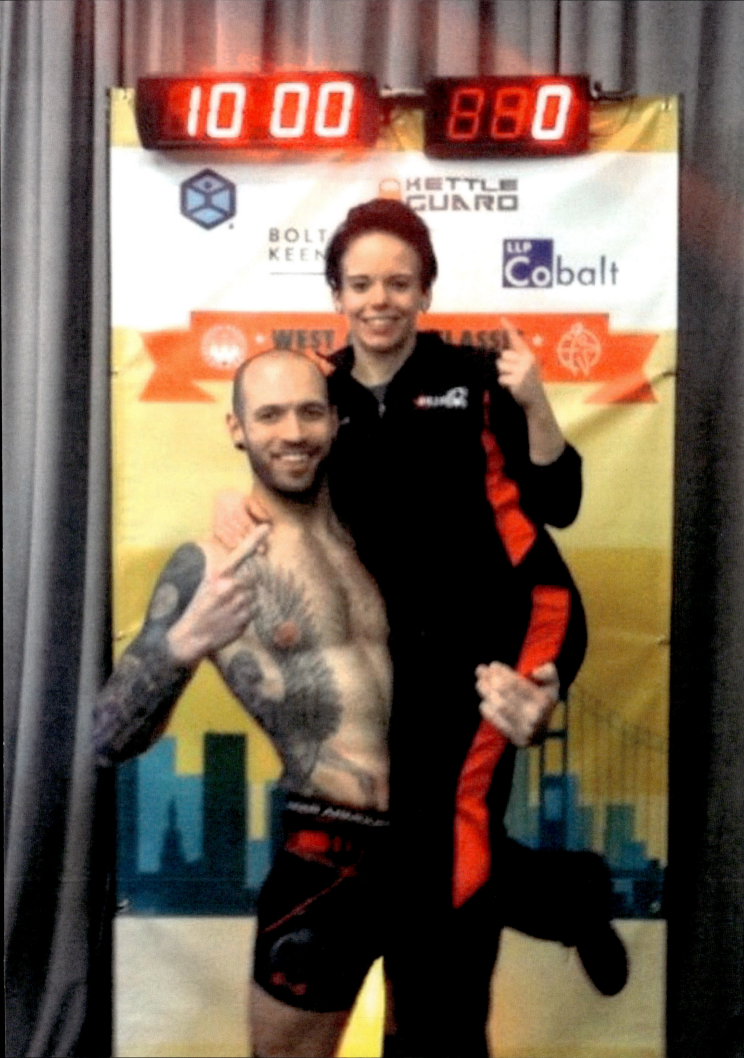

Weeks 5-8

Monday
1 x 8:00 Long Cycle

(With competition weight. If this is your first competition you may need to work up to this, in this first two weeks try to hit 6:00 in week 5 and then 7:00 in week 6 and then in weeks 7 and 8 you need to be hitting 8:00. Try to maintain 5rpm.)

4 Rounds:

10-15 Decline Push Ups
5-10 Pull Ups or Reverse (Suspension/TRX) Rows

Finish:

5 sets of alternating 2:00 Row and 2:00 Run

Tuesday
3 sets of static 0:30 one arm overhead holds on each arm with one step up from comp weight

5 Rounds Lifting:

5 Squats (Front or Back Squats, your preference)
10 Chin Ups
5 BB Deadlift
10 Skull Crushers or Band Pull Downs or Tricep

Finish: 10k bike ride or 10 x 1:00/0:20 intervals on Airdyne and Box Steps (20:00 total)

Wednesday
1 x 2:00 Double Cleans (one step below comp weight)

6 x 2:00/1:00 Rounds Long Cycle
(Do the first 3 rounds with comp weight and then 3 rounds with one step down. The goal here is decent speed, not quite a sprint but close. You still need to perform good lockouts and fixate properly, but you need to spend as little time in rack as possible.)

1 x 3:00 Jerks (One step below comp weight at 8rpm.)

3 Sets of:
5 BB Shoulder presses (take at least 60 seconds between sets)
0:30 Seated Grip Drill: on a bench, legs wide, back straight, two kettlebells, swing just a couple inches back and forth, using two steps up from comp weight.

10 x 1:00/0:15 Rounds of cardio interval work (running, jumping rope, bike, boxing, etc)

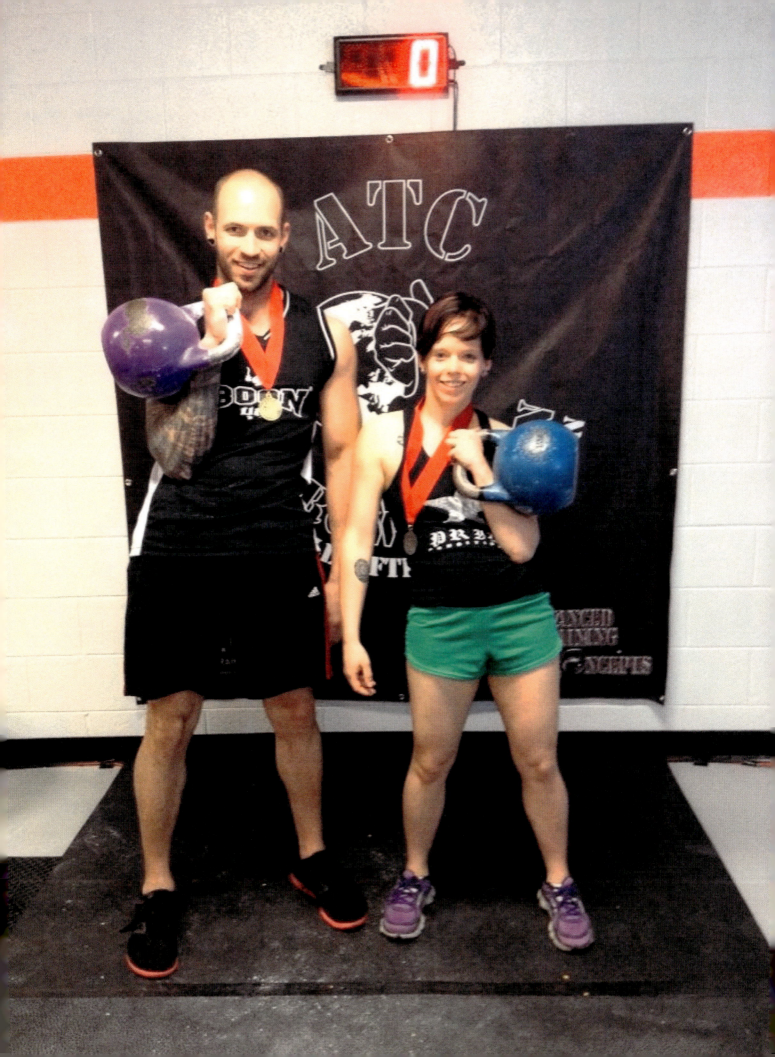

Weeks 5-8

Thursday
Cardiac Development

3 x 3:00 x 4 sets (total work time is 36:00)
-Row
-Run
-AMRAP: 3 Burpees, 3 Jump Squats, 30 Mountain Climbers
There is no rest in this workout, your pace will be and should be slower!

Friday
8 x 1:00/0:30 Long Cycle Sprints (First 4 @ comp weight and then 4 @ one step down. Try to maintain 7-8rpm each round.)

Lifting:
5 Sets
-5 BB Back Squats
-10 DB Curls
-30 Half Jumps (Lower to half squat position like your first or second dip and EXPLODE!)
-10 Band Pull Downs or Rope Tricep Extensions

4 x 15 BB Quarter Squat Jumps (with 1:00 rest between sets)
*It is important that you land soft! If you do not land soft the bar will hurt you!
*Do not string together your jumps, make each jump as high as possible, land soft, rest by standing up straight, make your dip just like your first dip on Long Cycle and explode!
*Use a weight 20%-25% heavier than what you will push in competition

Sprints:
10 x 30 Meter sprints with 0:30 rest between each sprint

Saturday
Lifting:

5 Sets
-5 Deadlifts
-5 BB Shoulder Press
-10 Glute Ham Raise
-10 Skull Crushers

Finish:

3 x 5:00 Jump Rope or Boxing/Kickboxing or 15:00 Run or Row

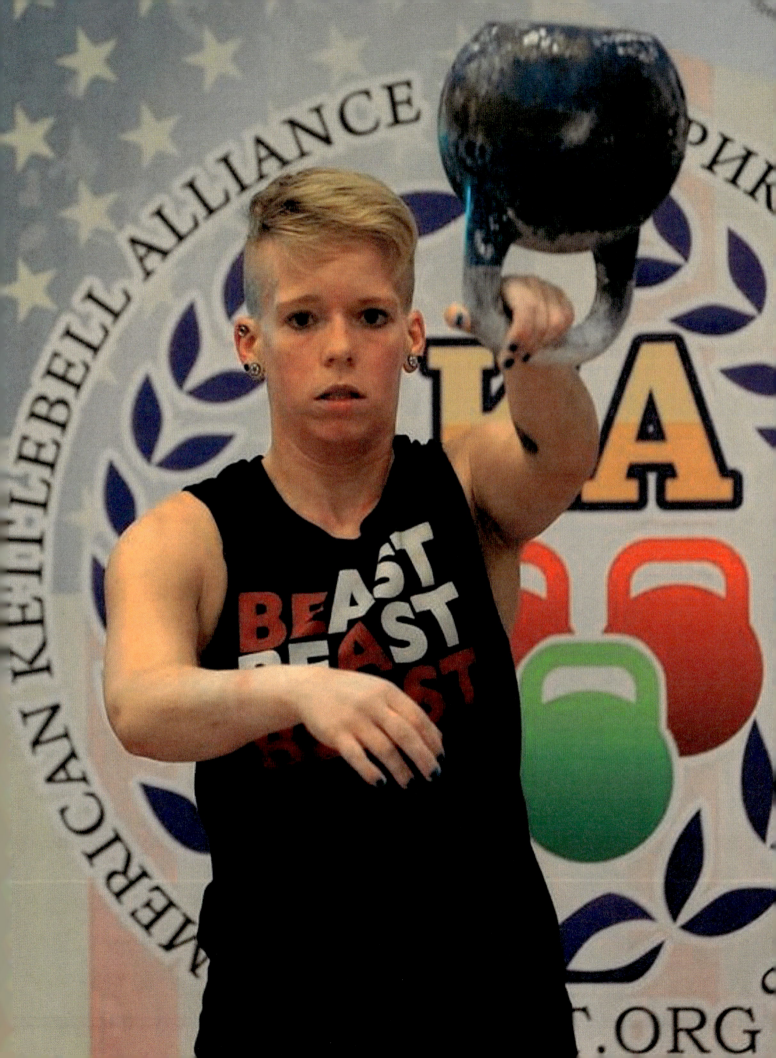

Weeks 9-12

I am not going to lie to you or sugar coat this, the last four weeks of this program are miserable but you will survive and you will make astonishing gains in your lifting during this time. You will hurt and you will be sore but it will all be worth it!

Monday – A Week
1 x 8:00 Long Cycle

(With competition weight! Try to alternate between 6rpm and 5rpm every other minute. On weeks 10 and 12 I want you to make a 10:00 set on alternating pace.)

3 Rounds:

10-15 Decline Push Ups
5-10 Pull Ups or Reverse (Suspension/TRX) Rows

Finish:

2 sets of alternating 5:00 Row and 5:00 Run (total work time is 20:00)

Tuesday
Kettlebell:

3 x 2:00on/2:00off LC (With comp weight)

3 x 0:30/0:30 Static Overhead Hold with one step up from comp weight (1:00 rest)

3 Rounds Lifting:
5 Squats (Front or Back Squats, your preference)
10 Chin Ups

Finish: 10k bike ride or 10 x 1:00/0:20 intervals on Airdyne and Box Step Jumps (20:00 total)

Wednesday

10 x 1:00/0:15 Rounds of cardio interval work (running, jumping rope, bike, boxing, etc)

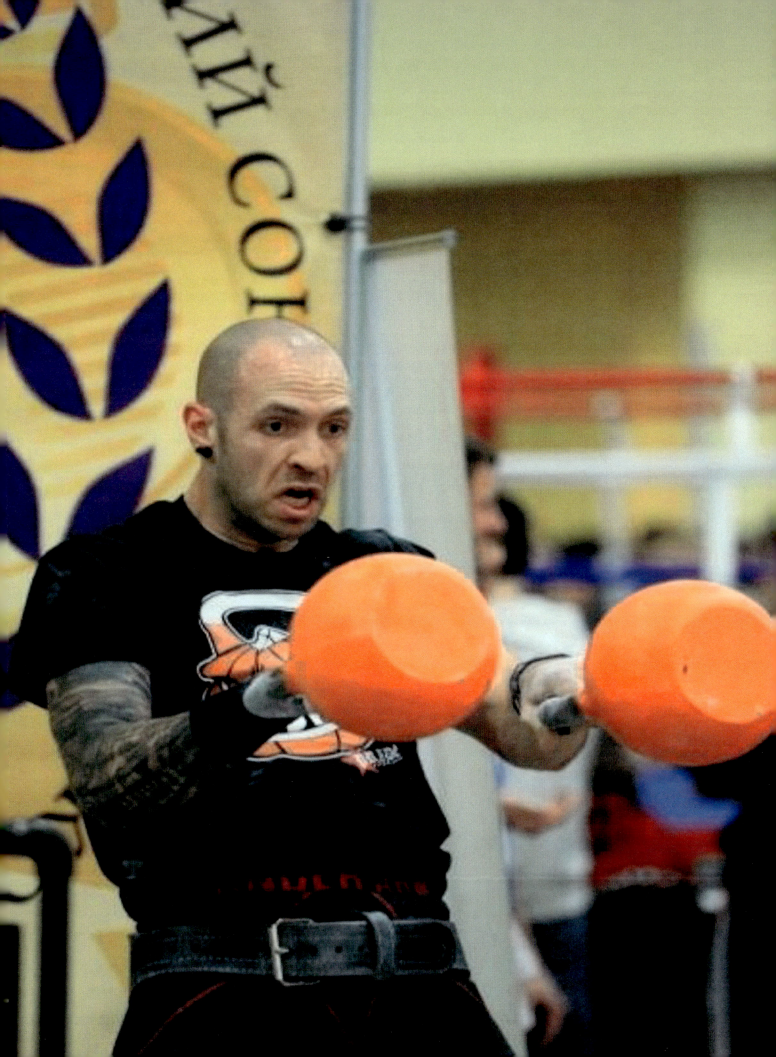

Weeks 9-12

Thursday
Kettlebell:

1 x 6:00 (With comp weight at one RPM faster than your 10:00 pace)

Cardiac Development
2 x 3:00
-Row
-Run
-AMRAP: 3 Burpees, 3 Jump Squats, 30 Mountain Climbers
There is no rest in this workout, your pace will be and should be slower!

Friday
1 x 2:00 Cleans with comp weight

8 x 1:00/0:30 Long Cycle Sprints (First 6 sets @ comp weight, last 4 sets at one step down. Try to maintain 8rpm all rounds.)

1 x 4:00 Jerks (With one step down from comp weight at 8rpm.)

Lifting:
3 Sets
-5 BB Back Squats + 5 Quarter Squat Jumpers
-10 DB Curls
-10 Band Pull Downs or Rope Tricep Extensions

4 x 25 BB Quarter Jumps
*It is important that you land soft! If you do not land soft the bar will hurt you!
*Do not string together your jumps, make each jump as high as possible, land soft, rest by standing up straight, make your dip just like your first dip on Long Cycle and explode!
*Use a weight 20%-25% heavier than what you will push in competition

3 x 1 mile repeats with 2:00 break then 5 x 30 Meter sprints with 0:30 rest between each sprint

Saturday
Lifting:

3 Sets
-5 Deadlifts
-5 BB Shoulder Press
-10 Glute Ham Raise
-10 Skull Crushers

Finish:
4 x 5:00 Jump Rope or Boxing/Kickboxing or 20:00 Run or Row

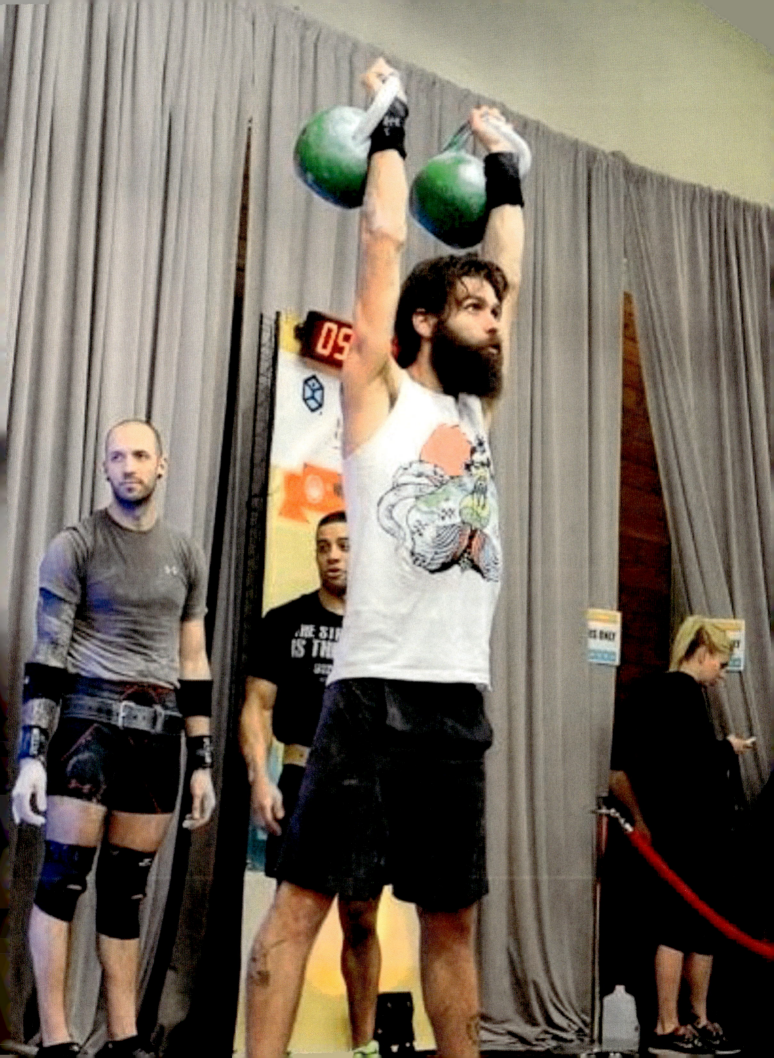

Week 13 – Competition Week!

This week is what is known in the competition world as "tapering". Whether you are a fighter, a distance runner, triathlete, power-lifter, etc, all of these athletes taper their training on the week before competition. You are now an athlete and you will taper too. So here is your competition week...

Monday – A Week
1 x 8:00 Long Cycle

(With competition weight! Try to maintain 6rpm.)

Finish:

2 sets of alternating 5:00 Row and 5:00 Run (total work time is 20:00)

Tuesday
3 Rounds Lifting:

5 Squats (Front or Back Squats, your preference)
5 Chin Ups

Finish: 10:00 bike ride or run

Wednesday
Kettlebell:

3 x 2:00/2:00 LC (First set at comp weight, second one step down and third two steps down)
1 x 2:00 Jerks (On comp weight at 10rpm)

1 x 5:00 round of cardio (jumping rope, bike, etc)

Thursday
Cardio:

1 x 10:00
-Row or Run (nothing hard or fast, nice easy pace just to break a sweat and loosen up. If you are traveling on this day then try to get your row or run in the morning before you leave and then relax when you get to your destination. If you are stiff from traveling, go for a one mile walk when you get to your competition destination.)

Friday
Do nothing! Rest! You may be traveling on this day and you may be going to weigh ins. Get in a decent walk around one or two miles and then stretch for 30 minutes. I do not recommend cutting weight for your first comp to make a certain weight class, don't worry about it and just go have fun!

Saturday
Eat a huge breakfast and go compete and kick ass!

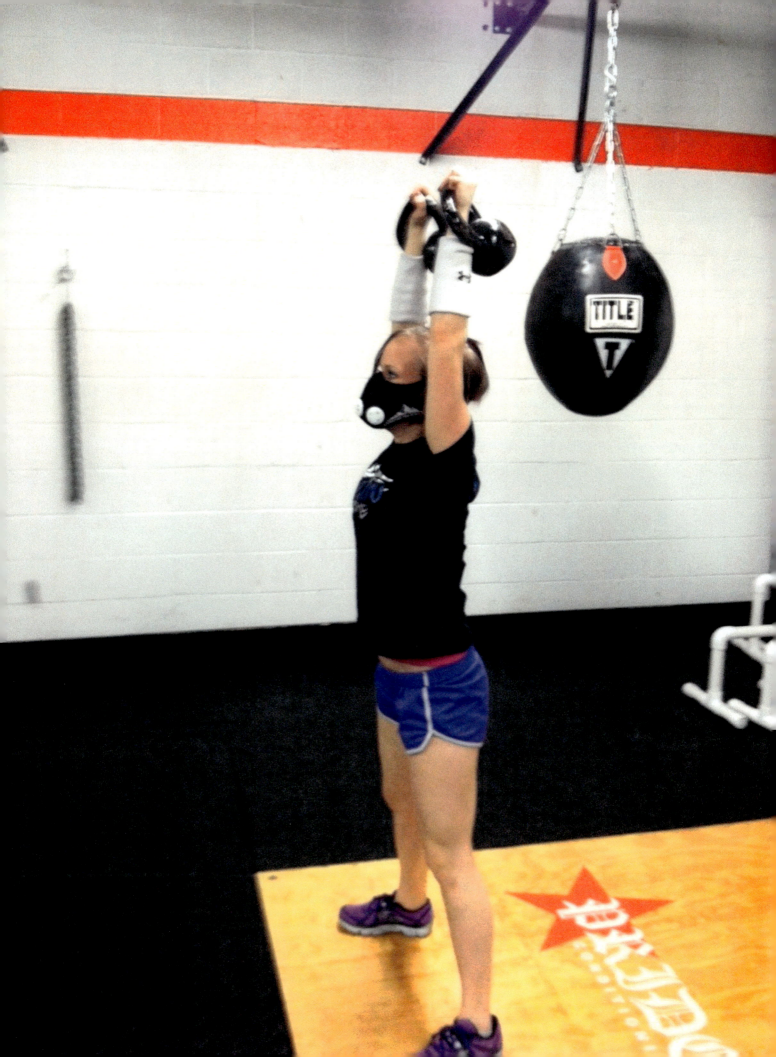

Training Mask

While the "Elevation Training Mask" is not essential to this program, I must write something about its use and the benefits of use. The Elevation Training Mask simulates the lack of oxygen at altitudes above sea level. We (my wife Lindsay and I) have used the mask ourselves during fight training and we use it during kettlebell training as well. I do not recommend using the mask everyday, maybe every other week, once a week at the most. I suggest doing some of your finish cool down/burnout cardio work after your kettlebell sets with the mask on. You can also go for shorter runs with the mask on, although it may terrify people on the sidewalk and driving by in their cars!

The essential part of training with the mask is not just the lack of oxygen while you are working, but the real magic and benefit comes from the lack of oxygen on your breaks or recovery time. Getting use to working with less oxygen and trying to recover on your breaks with less oxygen is difficult to say the least, and you will feel the benefits of training with the mask. Do be aware that the mask takes some getting used to, and if you are claustrophobic or get anxious easily, the mask will scare you, but stay calm, you'll be fine, you won't die or pass out, I promise! Part of training with the mask and it's benefit is getting used to that out of breath feeling and the "fight or flight" panic response that comes with it, once you can overcome this response and learn to stay calm, keep your heart rate and your breathing under control, you will start pushing through kettlebell sets like a machine!

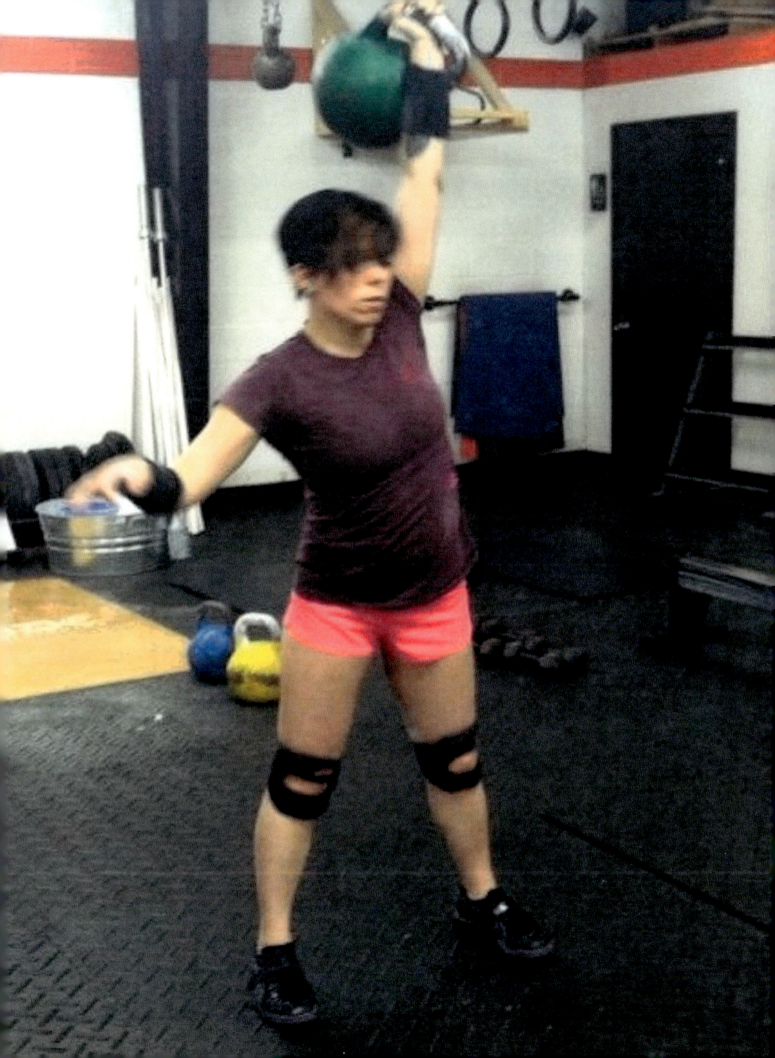

Recovery

Post-workout always be sure to stretch out your hands, forearms and legs. Also be sure to use a foam roller and/or a "Tiger Tail" to massage out all the lactic acid in your muscles. A tip for stretching fingers; use a rubber band or two from bunches of broccoli or asparagus. Place your fingers inside the rubber band and spread your fingers out, repeat, a lot, on both hands for a total of around 5 minutes on each hand. Our other favorite hand stretch is actually for your forearms and you simply go down to the ground on all fours, then externally rotate your hands back towards your knees and stay in that position for 60 seconds, repeat if needed.

Another great recovery is obviously stretching, but sometimes we don't know how to properly stretch, which muscles to stretch, how long to hold, etc. To solve all of your stretching questions and misdirection, seek out a "Deep Stretch" class at a yoga studio. In a deep stretch class you will be directed and physically assisted in your stretches by qualified and certified instructors. In most deep stretch classes you will hold the stretch for about 3 minutes, which will allow your muscles and joints to truly relax and stretch out a little farther. Too much of a good thing is, well, not good, so I do not recommend going to a hot deep stretch class, the heat in these classes claim the benefit of allowing you to stretch even deeper than you would at a normal 70 degree room while they have heat turned up to around 90-100 degrees. Stretching deeper in the heat is, in my personal and professional opinion, not good for your muscles or joints and I have personally witnessed several of my clients try a hot deep stretch class and come back injured and unable to train for weeks.

I also highly recommend seeking out a professional rehab and/or physical therapist. A qualified physical therapist will do movement tests to check your mobility and they can direct you to specific exercises and stretches to increase your mobility and strengthen your stabilizer muscles, which will in turn allow you to push harder and faster without injury. The greatest thing I can recommend is to find a physical therapist who has been trained in a therapy method called "Trigger Point Dry Needling" or just "Dry Needling" for short. This method of therapy uses an acupuncture needle and breaks up knots in your soft tissue that may be preventing you from moving properly or achieving proper mobility. I can tell you from experience that this method is both highly effective and will give you immediate results in just one session, as opposed to other methods of therapy that require multiple sessions (I go to get needled once a month). I tell my clients who inquire about dry needling that it is 10 times more effective than a deep tissue massage and takes 1/10 the time. Find a therapist that does dry needling and go be a pin cushion for ten minutes, the benefits are simply amazing. If you are having knee pains from Long Cycle or from running or squatting, or if you cannot straighten your arms in a good lockout, getting needled will help you, I promise!

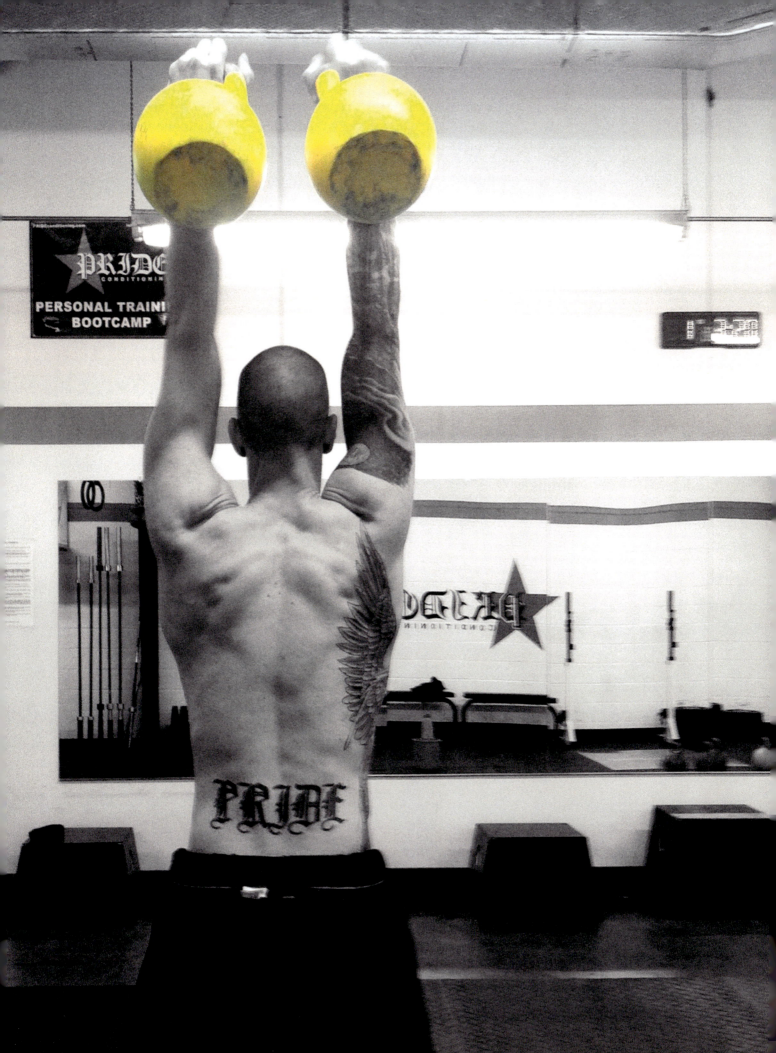

VO2 Max & Cardiac Development

You will also see a good deal of running or other cardio work in the program schedule. This is not only to increase cardio vascular output and increase VO2 max and lactic acid threshold, on top of maintaining weight, but it is also in the program as recovery. Running (in conjunction with stretching and rolling and drinking lots of water) will help flush out all the lactic acid that builds up in your legs with all the long cycle training and heavy squats and deadlifts and box jumps. The downside to running is the impact it has on the body; while it is one of the best forms of cardio, it is also one of the highest impact exercises you can do. Many people get into kettlebell training to stay away from high impact exercise; if you are one of those people you can substitute work on the Airdyne, an air rower, or stepmill, but nothing is as good as the real thing. I do not recommend running more than 3 miles as your long cycle set only takes 10 minutes and there is no point in working much past 2-3 times your competition time. In this program there are two types of cardio work, one its to push your heart rate to around 90% of it's max workload (usually between 165-185, this is VO2 max and lactic acid threshold development) and the other cardio work is a much slower heart rate (around 135 BPM this is cardiac development). The goal of VO2 max cardio work is to push your pace as fast as possible for a minimum of 10 minutes and a maximum of 20 minutes at the most. In order to increase your VO2 max threshold and your lactic acid threshold, this will get you used to the mental and physical exhaustion and torture of pushing hard for 10 minutes. The goal of cardiac development is to work at a pace that fills all four chambers of your heart completely before they contract, this will strengthen your heart muscle and the valves and chambers inside. Both of these methods of cardio work are specific in their heart rate zones, both are difficult in their own right.

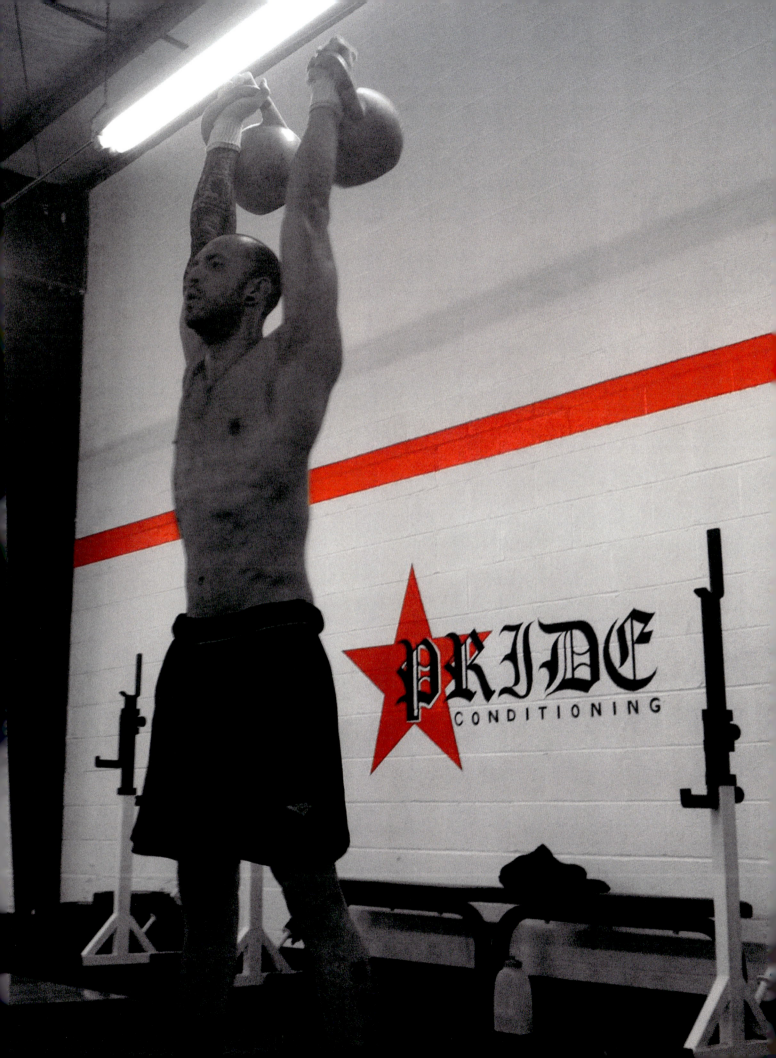

Diet During Training

If you are going to compete in a kettlebell competition you will be weighed in the morning of or the evening before the competition. With this in mind, you need to pick your weight class before you start. If this is your first competition I do not recommend cutting any weight, it is too much stress on the body and a huge amount of mental stress, and mental stress makes weight cutting very difficult. If you are going to cut weight to hit a certain weight class then I would not recommend cutting more than 5-10 pounds before your competition, unless you come from a wrestling or fighting background and you know how to properly cut weight and rehydrate. I have personally sabotaged my own performance cutting weight and I have seen many people cut weight too quickly without proper nutrition and hydration and their performance suffered greatly. Remember, weigh ins for kettlebell competitions are not always the day before the comp, a lot of them, especially smaller and more local comps are the morning of the competition. Be sure to double and triple check the date and time of weigh ins far in advance so you know when they are. Obviously if you have a day before weigh in then you can safely cut 5-10 pounds and put it back on, but if it is the morning of then you may have trouble doing this and again, unless you have experience cutting weight I do not recommend cutting any weight if this is your first competition.

If you insist on cutting weight to make a certain weight class then I will give you some pointers. It is very difficult to train for a competition and cut weight at the same time, you will be tired, angry, irritable, and your performance could suffer. I recommend not trying to cut weight until you are two to three weeks out, if you can maintain a very strict diet then you should be able to cut 5 pounds during the last week of training and then another 2-5 pounds in water weight the night before and morning of the competition. You need to measure all your food and track your calories. I would maintain just enough calories for the entire training program and then cut about 100 calories two weeks out and then 200 calories per day the week of. If you want to cut water weight (I am not going to go into great detail on cutting water weight), you need to over-hydrate for 48 hours before the competition, then the night before the event, cut your water down to only half what you were drinking the previous two days, and then the morning of, only a few sips of water or coffee and then nothing until weigh ins and no food (assuming weigh ins are before 12 noon, if they are after 12 then you can have a few more sips of water more frequently until the afternoon weigh in). Everyone and every body cuts water differently so I cannot promise it will work great for you and I cannot promise if it does work that you will completely rehydrate in time. Once you weigh in, I would have some energy bars, some fruit (high water content like melon or high sugar content like pineapple) and gatorade on hand and start chowing down and getting those fluids in. Be sure to go to the bathroom before you get on the platform, after slightly dehydrating and then having a mass amount of fluids and carbs you don't want to have an accident while lifting!

For your diet during training, you need a balance of carbs, protein and good fats. Stay clear of white bread and white potatoes. White bread will give you cramps and possibly shin splints. I also highly recommend anyone in the sports world avoid dairy like the plague, it will clog all of your systems and lungs and your organ cavity with mucus and your cardio vascular capacity and output will suffer.

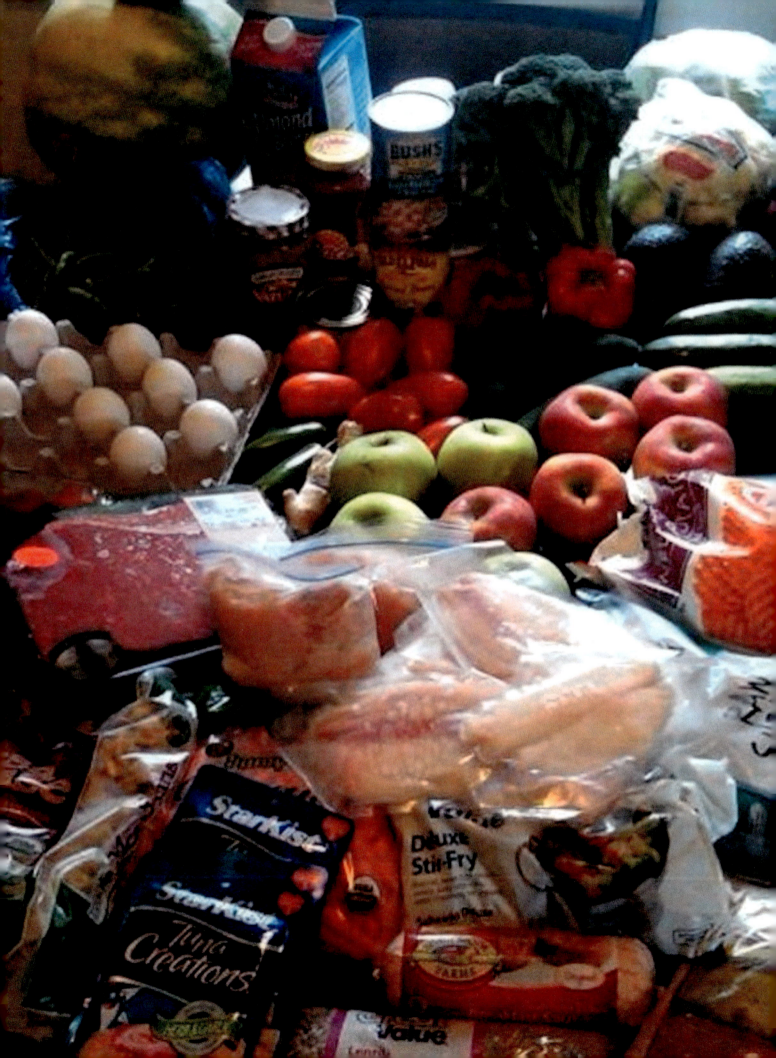

I recommend a protein shake (dairy- and animal-free mixed with almond milk) and half a banana an hour before your workout and the same an hour after along with two to three rice cakes to replenish your carb stores. Then you need a meal of solid food an hour or two after your post workout shake.

Basically, your diet should be composed of: lots of veggies, protein from lean meats like chicken and turkey, eggs, fish, healthy carbs like brown rice and sweet potato and good fats from coconut oil, olive oil and avocado. I also recommend staying away from wheat and gluten and anything processed and especially anything with sugar or HFCS (high fructose corn syrup) added to it.

The last thing I will highly recommend is Intermittent Fasting. In the sports nutrition world we are always looking for the next big thing and IF is it. The 6 equally sized, smaller meals per day came from the body building world where they needed a constant stream of nutrients going to their muscles all day, this method of eating also helps people who have trouble regulating their metabolism and also people who have major issues with portion control. The only problem with this method of nutrition is that we as humans were not truly meant to eat like this, it is a product of the modern world and the availability of food. It is also time consuming (to prep all that food) and it is very tough to maintain that schedule with our hectic training and work schedules. With that said, I truly believe that where there is a will there is a way, if you want success badly enough you will find the time to prep all your food on the weekend for the coming week and you will find a way to stay on that eating schedule, but I know it is tough. The alternative is Intermittent Fasting (IF), where you have a large window (12-14 hours) where you do not eat (but you can consume some liquids like coffee and water) and then you have a widow of time that you can eat (the remaining 10-12 hours). The basic theory behind IF is that hundreds of years ago, people did not eat much while roaming for game to kill or while picking berries from the woods, they usually got little to no food for a long period of the day and then were lucky to have one or two larger meals. Now a lot of people will argue this method of eating and say "you cannot process more than 300 calories of food at a time and any excess is stored as fat". Well, IF claims, that you are burning that stored fat during your fasting window! My wife and I and several of our clients use IF, we try not to eat after 9 PM and then we do not eat again until 9 or 10 or 11 AM, also, our first meal or two is not solid, it is a nutrient dense shake of plant based proteins, almond milk, fruit and almond butter for some good fats. Also, current research has shown that avoiding fats all together, will make you fat, as your body will hold onto and not burn its fat stores because it thinks it is not going to get anymore fat anytime soon. In our window of eating, we have our first two meals as liquid form with plant-based protein, then we have a balanced "real whole-food" meal, then one more plant based protein shake with a banana but without almond butter (because many believe that consuming fat post-workout will inhibit protein absorption), then we have one balanced meal of real whole-food for dinner and then we are done for the day and the window closes until the next day. Once the window is closed you cannot eat until the next window, so no midnight snacking!

Blatant product endorsement here...

If you are looking for a great pre-workout meal, meal replacement, or a great snack for when you are on the go, in the gym, out hiking or out on any city or backcountry adventure, please go check out the most amazing raw protein and energy bars in the world, CAVEBARS! You can order directly from the website at http://www.cavebars.com. Cavebars are all natural, raw, dairy soy gluten and animal free and are vegan! Full of organic ingredients, high calorie with good carbs and fats and no added sugar and no artificial ingredients or artificial sweeteners, these bars pack the energy and fuel you need.

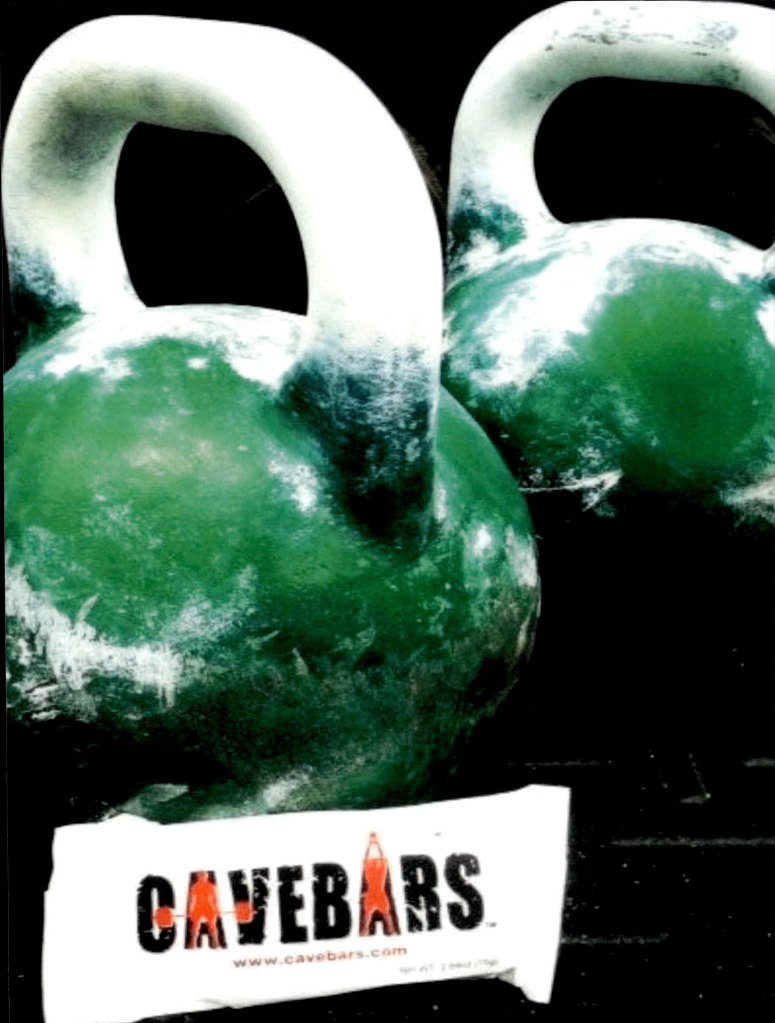

Doug's Vegan High Energy High Protein Shake Recipe

Here is my recipe for an amazing plant based protein smoothie that is easy to make, has ingredients you can get year round and above all it tastes amazing! (you can also read the full IF article and get more info on this recipe by [clicking here or going to this address http://prideconditioning.com/intermittent-fasting-101-the-team-seamans-smoothie-recipe/](http://prideconditioning.com/intermittent-fasting-101-the-team-seamans-smoothie-recipe/)):

20oz almond milk
1 apple
1.5 cups frozen tropical fruit (Lindsay uses frozen mixed berries)
2 big handfuls of spinach
1 cup frozen strawberries
2 tablespoons almond butter
2 scoops Plantfusion (soy free, dairy free, vegan protein powder)

Directions:

Pour almond milk into blender, add everything else, blend on high for three minutes. Done! Makes two 20oz shakes, I have one at 9am or so and the next at 12:00pm or so, about 60 minutes before I workout.

Here is the nutritional breakdown (per shake, remember this recipe makes two shakes):

calories: 448
carbs: 49g
fat: 17g
protein: 29g
sodium: 691g
sugar: 35g

I am 195 pounds and I am 75" tall. I have a decent amount of mass, and I workout everyday at a very high intensity, so I need to feed that mass and have enough energy stores for workouts, that is why this shake is this size. If you are smaller than me, you need to decrease this recipe accordingly, for example, Lindsay's shake is 1/3 less than mine. If you are bigger than me, but you are looking to lose weight, this size shake is perfect for you. And another note, this shake is for pre-workout meals, because it has fat in it, I have another shake after workout but it is just protein and a smaller amount of carbs, no fat, studies have proven that fat intake post-workout will inhibit protein uptake into the muscles.

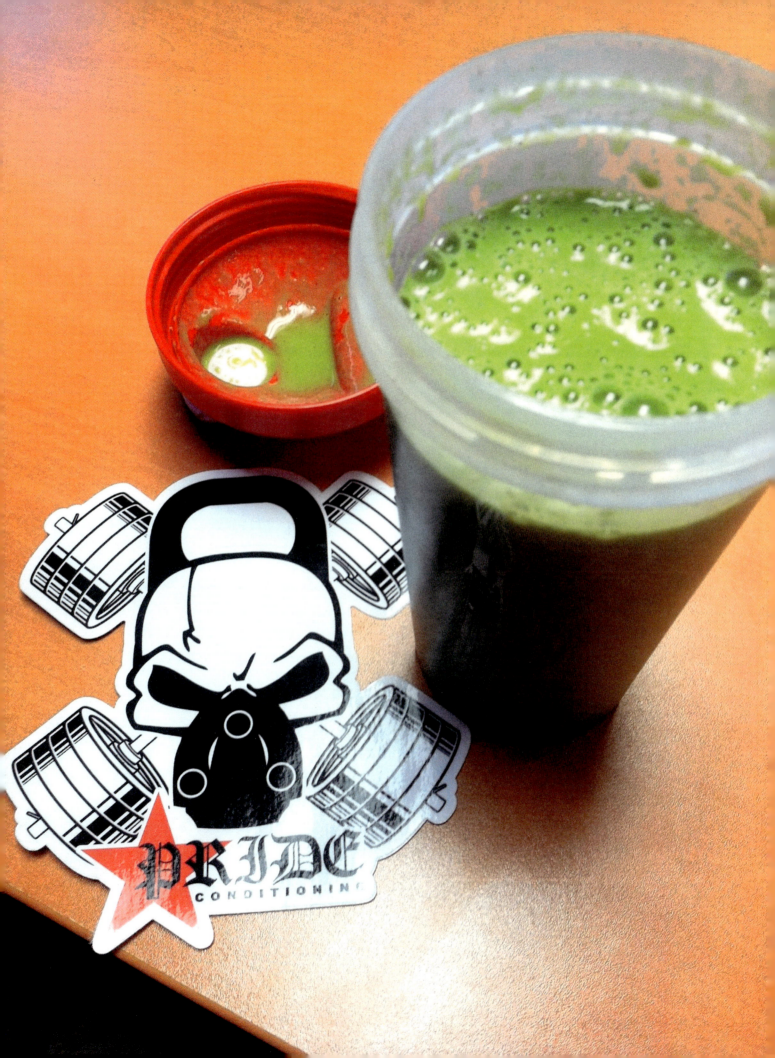

Conclusion and Thanks

I would like to thank you for taking the time to read this manual! I sincerely hope that the information in this manual will help you and if this is your very first competition it absolutely should help you, in fact I guarantee it will. If you have already competed then this manual may give you some different methods of training and possibly open your eyes to our way of doing things and it may help you train others to compete, but as I said at the very beginning, this manual is for beginners and first time competitors and is not geared towards or meant for experienced lifters. There are many methods of training and programming and this is just one, I do not claim this program and training method to be better than every other program in the world, but I promise you if this is your first competition it will improve your numbers. And if you are training without a coach this book will most certainly improve your numbers.

As I have stated many times throughout this book, if you are training on your own, please find a qualified coach to at least review your technique and give you some critiques on your technique and tips to improve it. If you have a good work ethic and train daily on the program I have laid out for you in this book, then you only need a coach to watch one or two of your sets each week or every other week and then spend the next week or two working on the tips that your coach gives you. If you cannot find a coach locally or the ones you find will only train you on a continuous or long term schedule, please email me at kettlebelltraining@prideconditioning.com and I will setup a video review with you.

You can also visit GSplanet.com for a complete list of all AKA/IUKL approved gyms and coaches as well as a list of rules, regulations, rankings tables and sanctioned competitions. This is the home site for the American Kettlebell Alliance, which is the American branch of the largest and oldest kettlebell organization in the world, the IUKL (International Union of Kettlebell Lifting). There are many other organizations and governing bodies promoting kettlebell sport but the IUKL is the largest and oldest and it is sanctioned by the Russian Sports Commission.

Kettlebell Sport is not for the faint of heart or the weak and it is especially not for the weak-minded. You are about to embark on a training regimen that requires a massive amount of discipline and dedication, I wish you the best of luck! I am confident you can accomplish any goal, but in the end you need to be confident and believe in yourself, so get out there, pick up those kettlebells and get your ass to work!

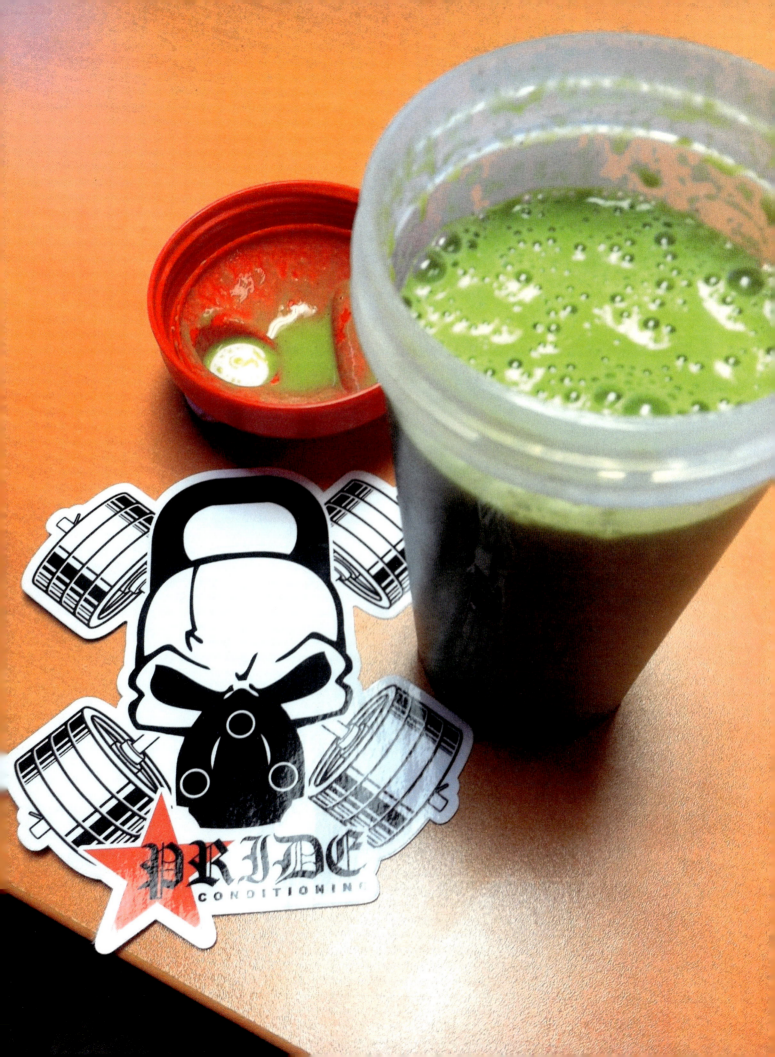

Conclusion and Thanks

I would like to thank you for taking the time to read this manual! I sincerely hope that the information in this manual will help you and if this is your very first competition it absolutely should help you, in fact I guarantee it will. If you have already competed then this manual may give you some different methods of training and possibly open your eyes to our way of doing things and it may help you train others to compete, but as I said at the very beginning, this manual is for beginners and first time competitors and is not geared towards or meant for experienced lifters. There are many methods of training and programming and this is just one, I do not claim this program and training method to be better than every other program in the world, but I promise you if this is your first competition it will improve your numbers. And if you are training without a coach this book will most certainly improve your numbers.

As I have stated many times throughout this book, if you are training on your own, please find a qualified coach to at least review your technique and give you some critiques on your technique and tips to improve it. If you have a good work ethic and train daily on the program I have laid out for you in this book, then you only need a coach to watch one or two of your sets each week or every other week and then spend the next week or two working on the tips that your coach gives you. If you cannot find a coach locally or the ones you find will only train you on a continuous or long term schedule, please email me at kettlebelltraining@prideconditioning.com and I will setup a video review with you.

You can also visit GSplanet.com for a complete list of all AKA/IUKL approved gyms and coaches as well as a list of rules, regulations, rankings tables and sanctioned competitions. This is the home site for the American Kettlebell Alliance, which is the American branch of the largest and oldest kettlebell organization in the world, the IUKL (International Union of Kettlebell Lifting). There are many other organizations and governing bodies promoting kettlebell sport but the IUKL is the largest and oldest and it is sanctioned by the Russian Sports Commission.

Kettlebell Sport is not for the faint of heart or the weak and it is especially not for the weak-minded. You are about to embark on a training regimen that requires a massive amount of discipline and dedication, I wish you the best of luck! I am confident you can accomplish any goal, but in the end you need to be confident and believe in yourself, so get out there, pick up those kettlebells and get your ass to work!

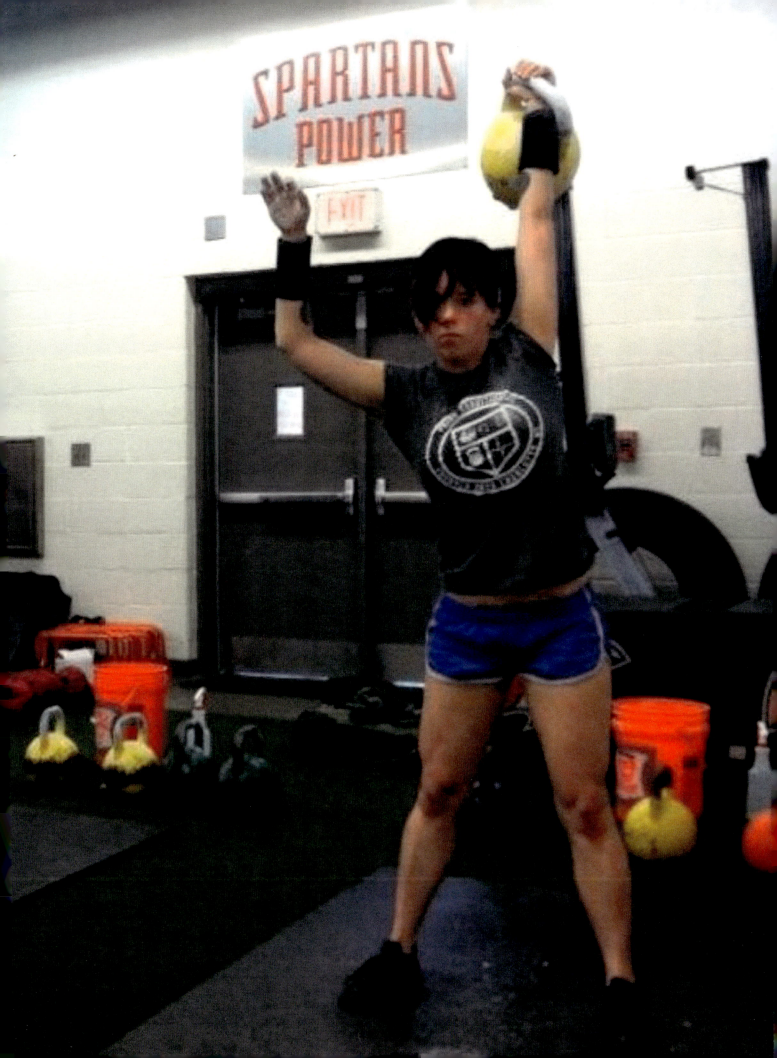

Made in the USA
Las Vegas, NV
11 May 2022

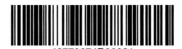